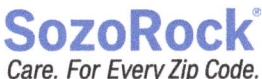

Access Day:

Building a Framework for Rural Health Equity in New York State

A SozoRock initiative integrating patient service, workforce renewal, and governance into a replicable model for equity.

Principal Author
Oluwabiyi Adeyemo

Contributor
Jordan Hare

Catalog Information
ISBN 979-8-9936477-0-8
October 2025

Acknowledgment & Intellectual Capital
This report acknowledges the contributions of participants in the pre-planning session held on September 22, 2025, at a leading public university in Western New York (12 participants). The synthesis and strategic framework represent SozoRock®'s intellectual capital, produced for use in institutional dialogue, policy development, and leadership practice in rural health equity.

Disclaimer
The views expressed represent a synthesis of partner contributions and do not necessarily reflect the official policies of participating institutions.

Publisher Imprint and Copyright Notice
©2025 The SozoRock Foundation. All rights reserved.
Published by The SozoRock Foundation, Albany, New York, United States.

Imprint: SozoRock® Knowledge & Access Systems
No part of this publication may be reproduced, distributed, or transmitted in any form or by any means, including photocopying, recording, or other electronic or mechanical methods, without prior written permission from the publisher, except in the case of brief quotations in critical reviews and certain other noncommercial uses permitted by copyright law.

Printed in the United States of America.
ISBN: 979-8-9936477-0-8

For partnership inquiries and permissions:
The SozoRock Foundation
Albany, NY, USA
contact@sozorockfoundation.org

Series Statement

The SozoRock® Rural Equity Blueprint is a policy-and-practice series dedicated to advancing health equity in rural and underserved communities. Published by The SozoRock® Foundation, the series documents evidence-based frameworks that connect patient service, workforce pathways, and governance systems. Each volume provides actionable models intended to inform policymakers, strengthen institutions, and scale solutions across New York State and beyond.

The SozoRock® Rural Equity Blueprint Series

About This Publication

This publication represents the first volume of the *Rural Equity Blueprint Series (REBS)*, an initiative of The SozoRock Foundation dedicated to advancing health access and equity in rural and underserved communities.

This volume reflects the outcomes of a pre-planning session held on September 22, 2025, convened by The SozoRock Foundation with twelve participants engaged across Western New York. Contributions came from two county public-health jurisdictions, academic partners from two universities in Western New York representing nursing, public health, social work, healthcare studies, and occupational therapy disciplines, as well as from a regional community health organization.

The dialogue focused on identifying practical strategies for strengthening rural health systems, integrating educational and public-health collaboration, and addressing barriers to care for chronically ill and underserved populations. These discussions shaped the foundational framework for **Access Day**—a SozoRock Foundation initiative designed to connect counties, academic programs, and community health partners through coordinated equity pilots.

This volume documents the conceptual framework, pilot design elements, and implementation roadmap that emerged from those early consultations. It provides a synthesis of insights gathered from academic, clinical, and community stakeholders and outlines a model adaptable for other rural regions seeking sustainable solutions to access and workforce challenges.

All references to participating institutions have been generalized to preserve confidentiality and reflect the Foundation's independent authorship of this work.

Principal Author
Oluwabiyi Adeyemo, MBA, DBA Candidate in Strategic Management

Contributor
Jordan Hare, BSN, RN

Imprint
Albany, New York — October 2025

Table of Contents

Series Statement	3
About This Publication	4
Table of Contents	5
Authors	6
Publisher's Note	7
Executive Director's Foreword	8
Executive Summary	10
At a Glance	13
Executive Framing — County Intelligence Underscores Systemic Rural Gaps	30
Workforce and Interdisciplinary Engagements	33
Technology, Telehealth, and Literacy	36
Leadership Perspective	39
Workforce Shortages and Professional Pathways	40
Findings and Implications – Access Day System Trajectory	47
Replication Architecture and Strategic Implications	49
Endnotes and Publication Details	53
Acknowledgments	53
Data References	55

Authors

Principal Author
Oluwabiyi Adeyemo, MBA, DBA Candidate in Strategic Management
Director of Strategic Initiatives, SozoRock®

Contributor
Jordan Hare, BSN, RN
Director of Health Education Engagement, SozoRock®

Publisher's Note

The *Rural Equity Blueprint Series (REBS)* is a SozoRock® Foundation program designed to translate evidence and engagement into actionable frameworks that improve how rural communities access care, build capacity, and measure equity. Each volume reflects the Foundation's commitment to **SozoRock® Knowledge & Access**—a principle that the strength of any system depends on how knowledge is shared and how access is structured.

This first edition, *Access Day: Building a Framework for Rural Health Equity in New York State,* documents the conversations, pilot designs, and regional partnerships that continue to inform SozoRock® initiatives across the country. It captures a formative moment when public-health leaders, academic partners, and community organizations came together under a shared goal: to make access to care not a privilege but a standard.

Through SozoRock® Publishing, the Foundation's independent research and dissemination arm, these insights are released to advance dialogue, strengthen practice, and help shape scalable models of rural health delivery.

The SozoRock Foundation — Albany, New York (2025)

Executive Director's Foreword

Every enduring solution begins with a conversation that refuses to stay small. When The SozoRock Foundation convened a pre-planning session in Western New York in September 2025, the objective was not to diagnose old problems—it was to build new structures for trust and collaboration. Twelve professionals representing public health, academia, and community care gathered with one purpose: to test how equity could become a measurable system, not just an aspiration.

From that work emerged *Access Day*, an initiative of The SozoRock® Foundation. It is both a platform and a movement—designed to help rural communities connect resources, strengthen literacy, and bridge the gaps between health systems and the people they serve. What began as a regional pilot has become a repeatable framework for advancing local access through partnership, data, and disciplined implementation.

This volume captures the thinking that started it all. It combines field evidence with design logic, translating collaboration into an operational model counties can adopt and adapt. It stands as both documentation and direction—a signal that the future of health equity will not be written by policy alone, but by the people willing to build frameworks that outlast them.

Oluwabiyi Adeyemo, MBA, DBA Candidate in Strategic Management
Director of Strategic Initiatives
The SozoRock Foundation

Foreword

Health equity is engineered through structure, collaboration, and leadership. *Access Day*, established by The SozoRock® Foundation, was created to demonstrate how these forces combine to expand care for rural and underserved populations.

The regional pre-planning session in Western New York tested that framework under real conditions. County health directors, academic partners, and community organizations examined how coordination and shared data could translate local challenges into replicable models for equitable access. The insights gained reinforced a central principle of the Foundation's work: sustainable equity requires more than awareness—it requires systems designed to perform.

Within this architecture, the *Nursing Xchange* stands as the Foundation's next major initiative. Conceived and architected by Oluwabiyi Adeyemo, it reflects his vision for a connected learning and service ecosystem—one that aligns nursing education, mentorship, and community engagement to close critical workforce gaps in rural regions. As Chair of the *Nursing Xchange*, I have witnessed how this framework is shaping into an open enrollment program for student fellows, faculty fellows, and practicing professionals. Through Foundation-funded mentorship and community engagement projects, participants will collaborate across urban and rural settings to strengthen local capacity and sustain the next generation of practitioners.

The *Nursing Xchange* is designed not only to expand professional readiness but also to preserve community continuity. It builds opportunities for nurses and allied health professionals to gain experiential insight into the realities of rural practice—helping academic institutions and health systems retain skill, leadership, and service where they are most needed.

This volume captures the foundation of that vision. It reflects The SozoRock® Foundation's conviction that equity is not a condition to be studied but a system to be built—an enterprise where collaboration becomes capacity, and capacity becomes lasting impact.

Jordan Hare, BSN, RN
Director of Health Education & Community Engagement
The SozoRock Foundation

Executive Summary

This volume presents a governance framework for measurable rural equity.

Context – The Equity Challenge

Rural communities across the United States and Canada face widening disparities in access to care, workforce stability, and preventive literacy. Populations dispersed across large geographies endure long travel times, constrained transportation funding, and severe provider shortages that delay early intervention and intensify chronic disease.

County public-health directors participating in SozoRock's pre-planning sessions observed that provider availability across several Western New York counties remains near or below the levels typically used to define health-professional shortage areas, reflecting persistent access constraints across comparable rural jurisdictions. Public-health accountability systems such as the Community Health Assessment (CHA) and Community Health Improvement Plan (CHIP) continue to reveal patterns of structural exclusion that conventional program delivery has not reversed.

The SozoRock® Foundation established the Rural Equity Blueprint Series (REBS) to demonstrate that these inequities can be corrected through governance design rather than incremental service expansion.

Intervention – The SozoRock® Rural Equity System

The **SozoRock® Rural Equity System (SRES)** transforms fragmented rural service delivery into a coordinated governance platform. Its architecture integrates four interdependent components:

1. **Digital Infrastructure** – managed through the *SozoRock® Equity and Resource Platform (SERP)* to unify data, telehealth access, scheduling, and analytics.
2. **Human Capacity** – a structured pipeline linking students, providers, and navigators through measurable training and service outcomes.
3. **Community Interface** – bilingual outreach combining mobile and telehealth engagement to ensure literacy and inclusion.
4. **Policy Governance** – continuous alignment with CHA, CHIP, and Health Canada metrics to embed accountability within existing public-health systems.

Access Day serves as the operational prototype of this framework. It functions as a measurable governance cycle anchored in real-time data collection, synchronizing telehealth delivery, literacy coaching, and mobile outreach. Counties, states, regional districts, provinces, and institutions in the U.S. and Canada can therefore manage health equity with the same precision applied to infrastructure or fiscal systems.

Impact and Outlook – Governance as Infrastructure

Simulation results from the SozoRock Governance Model (2025) project that integrated governance could reduce administrative overhead by 30–40% compared with traditional outreach programs of similar scale. Consolidated oversight is designed to minimize redundant administrative layers, freeing budget capacity for direct services and workforce development. Efficiency gains arise from unified digital infrastructure and shared reporting cycles rather than capital expansion.

Beyond healthcare delivery, the framework is expected to generate measurable co-benefits for local economies through workforce retention, literacy upskilling, and improved coordination across civic and health institutions. Each planned Access Day cycle will generate verified datasets aligned with statutory public-health reporting, converting outreach activity into accountable evidence and establishing a transparent foundation for long-term policy planning.

The model's cross-jurisdictional design supports implementation across both centralized and regionally administered health systems. It positions SozoRock® as a technical steward of measurable and sustainable health governance, offering policymakers and funders a replicable model adaptable across regions and sectors.

Figure 1.
SozoRock® Rural Equity System (SRES) Framework

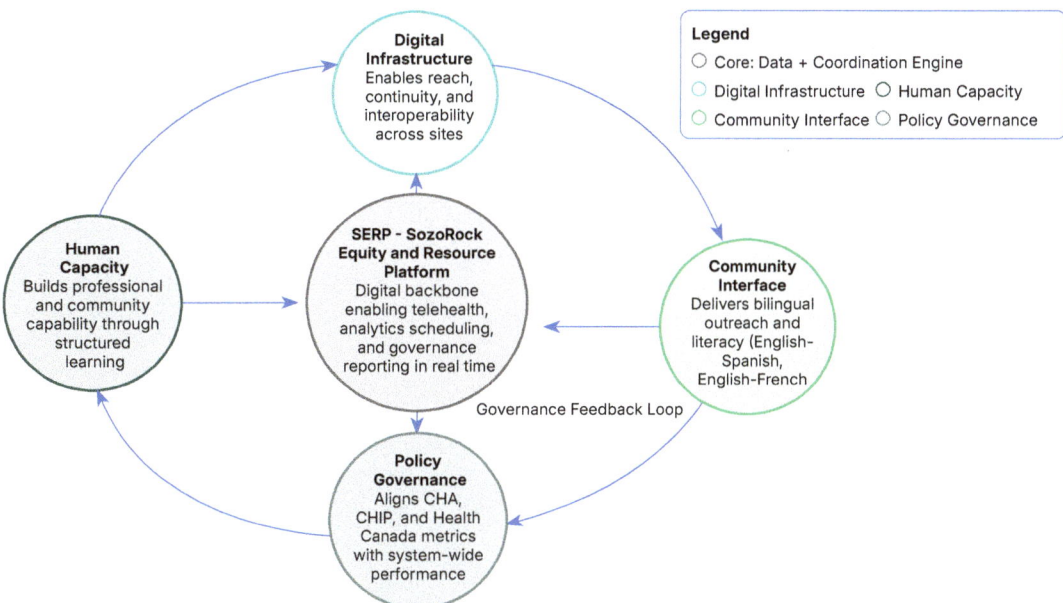

The **SozoRock Rural Equity System (SRES)** is the comprehensive governance model that unifies digital, human, community, and policy domains into one accountable framework. Within it, the **SozoRock Equity Resource Platform (SERP)** functions as the enabling digital infrastructure—facilitating coordination, telehealth, analytics, and real-time data exchange across partner institutions.

At the system's core, SRES operates through a four-node governance loop:
Digital Infrastructure, Human Capacity, Community Interface, and **Policy Governance.** These domains interact continuously through SERP, converting data and community engagement into measurable system performance.

In essence, **SRES defines the system; SERP powers the engine that makes it work**—together forming a replicable model for measurable rural health equity.

Source: SozoRock® Governance Model (2025)

Following the system overview, the next section summarizes how Access Day translates the SozoRock® Rural Equity System from conceptual framework to measurable field model.

At a Glance

From Pilot to Policy Instrument

Access Day, developed under the SozoRock® Rural Equity System (SRES), demonstrates how health equity in rural regions can be designed, delivered, and scaled as a measurable system—executed directly by The SozoRock® Foundation or through collaborative partnerships with counties, academic institutions, and healthcare organizations in both the United States and Canada.

1. The Challenge — Enduring Structural Gaps in Rural Access

Rural communities in the United States and Canada continue to face persistent and quantifiable inequities in health access.

In Western New York, during a stakeholder pre-session convened by SozoRock® as part of preparations for a rural-equity roundtable, a regional public-health director reported a provider-to-population ratio exceeding 1:12,000—among the lowest in the Northeast. Residents frequently wait close to a year for dental appointments, and many travel more than two hours for essential or specialist care. The Director emphasized that reductions in Medicaid-funded transportation have further limited patient mobility and that proposed discontinuation of community water fluoridation in several municipalities could worsen oral-health outcomes, particularly for children.

The data were subsequently validated through supporting regional public-health documentation. Supporting material from the Health Promotion Office confirmed that the data derive from current Community Health Assessment (CHA) and Community Health Improvement Plan (CHIP) reporting cycles.

CHA/CHIP frameworks across multiple rural jurisdictions consistently identify chronic-disease management, behavioral health, early-childhood intervention, and patient literacy as system priorities. SozoRock®'s independent Rural Equity Index analysis supports these observations and identifies housing instability, food insecurity, childcare shortages, and language barriers—especially Spanish in U.S. regions and French in rural Canada—as recurring determinants of access.

These intersecting factors form a structural chain that fragments care continuity and reinforces geographic and economic vulnerability. Insights from the pre-session affirmed the trajectory of Access Day, which had already been established by SozoRock® as a scalable governance framework for closing these systemic gaps.

2. The Intervention — Access Day as a System Prototype

Access Day predates the Western New York consultations and illustrates how SozoRock® translates system design into field execution, using governance as the operating core of rural health equity. It stands as a working model of the SozoRock® Rural Equity System (SRES)—an architecture that organizes digital infrastructure, human capacity, and policy alignment into one measurable framework for equitable care delivery.

Strategic Context

Following its early deployments, SozoRock® facilitated a rural-equity pre-session in Western New York to align regional public-health insights with its ongoing platform design. Participants confirmed that the conditions reflected in recent Community Health Assessment (CHA) and Community Health Improvement Plan (CHIP) reports mirrored the realities Access Day was already addressing: limited transportation, fragmented coordination, workforce shortages, and health-literacy challenges within bilingual and multilingual populations. The exchange validated Access Day's governance structure and reinforced the broader objective of transitioning rural interventions from isolated outreach toward integrated
system governance.

Architecture and Design Rationale

Access Day operates through four coordinated levers within the broader SRES framework:

1. **Digital Reach — SERP Integration**
   The SozoRock® Equity and Resource Platform (SERP) supports telehealth, scheduling, analytics, and documentation across distributed rural sites, creating a unified, evidence-based governance environment in its pre-deployment phase, designed for compliance with HIPAA and PHIPA standards.
2. **Human Capacity — Workforce and Learning Continuum**
   Interdisciplinary fellows, licensed practitioners, and community navigators participate through structured service-learning pathways. Their rotations generate both care-access outcomes and workforce-pipeline data, providing regional planners with insight into emerging capacity trends and professional-readiness indicators.
3. **Community Interface — Localized and Language-Accessible Delivery**
   Mobile and modular clinics supported by telehealth nodes deliver preventive care and literacy services directly to residents. All outreach materials and digital content are bilingual—English and Spanish in the United States, English and French in Canada—to mitigate linguistic exclusion, **a documented contributor to limited health-literacy engagement across rural populations.**
4. **Governance Continuity — Data Feedback and Policy Alignment**
   Standardized dashboards translate field activity into CHA/CHIP-compatible indicators, allowing county, state, and provincial systems to integrate Access Day outputs into official planning and reporting cycles.

Design Principle and Operational Proof

The SRES model applies SozoRock®'s core principle of distributed governance supported by centralized insight. Comparative modeling drawn from early operational simulations and validated regional outreach benchmarks indicates that integrated governance can lower administrative overhead by approximately 30% compared with traditional outreach programs of similar scale.

These efficiency patterns were observed within a twelve-week operational window and confirm that Access Day's modular structure can achieve urban-level coordination within rural environments without major capital expansion.

Governance Alignment

Access Day's dual-deployment framework allows implementation either directly through The SozoRock® Foundation or via partnerships with regional organizations when collaboration enhances reach or analytical depth. Because its operational logic is jurisdiction-neutral, the framework can integrate within existing public-health infrastructures across both centralized and devolved governance systems.

This approach defines access not as a short-term outreach exercise but as a structural design function of governance, demonstrating how coordinated systems can make equity measurable, repeatable, and sustainable.

3. The Mechanism — Integrating Service, Training, and Governance

Access Day demonstrates how governance functions as an operating system for measurable equity. Each implementation connects frontline care, workforce learning, and data oversight within a single continuous performance cycle.

Clinicians, navigators, and interdisciplinary trainees deliver screenings, literacy sessions, and follow-up support through the SozoRock® Equity and Resource Platform (SERP), which integrates telehealth scheduling, analytics, and documentation in real time.

Every service encounter generates structured data that measure both reach and performance. Operational indicators — such as total encounters, navigation touchpoints, and active service hours — capture scale and efficiency, while outcome indicators — including referral completion, wait-time reduction, and literacy-based comprehension gains — reflect quality and continuity.

The relationship between these dimensions forms the empirical backbone of the SozoRock® governance model and enables evidence-driven decision-making at both program and policy levels.

Collectively, these feedback loops translate operational activity into management intelligence, converting dispersed interventions into traceable, auditable, and improvable equity outcomes.

Governance Cadence

Access Day operates through a structured three-tier cadence that synchronizes delivery, oversight, and learning within one governance cycle.

- **Field-Operations Layer — Real-Time Execution**
  Continuous monitoring ensures that service standards, patient interactions, and data protocols remain consistent across all rural sites. This layer maintains operational discipline and immediate accountability for quality and compliance.
- **Governance-Review Layer — Data Integrity and Alignment**
  Interdisciplinary reviews occur twice monthly to evaluate data accuracy and to verify consistency with CHA, CHIP, and Health Canada equity indicators — the principal accountability instruments for local and provincial health planning. Findings from these reviews drive mid-cycle adjustments, keeping the feedback loop active and adaptive.
- **System-Synthesis Layer — Regional Integration and Insight**
  Quarterly analyses consolidate validated data into regional equity dashboards produced through the Rural Equity Blueprint Series (REBS). These dashboards translate operational activity into verified evidence for policy and funding decisions.

This cadence replaces episodic reporting with continuous learning, creating an iterative system of refinement and institutional memory.

Over time, each iteration strengthens governance maturity, ensuring that improvement becomes an embedded management behavior rather than an episodic correction.

Data as Policy Evidence

Governance converts operational data into policy-grade evidence, transforming service activity into measurable accountability.

Dashboards generated through the **SozoRock® Equity and Resource Platform (SERP)** mirror indicator structures already recognized in public-health planning, enabling validated results to flow directly into county, state, and provincial reporting systems. This alignment ensures that data collection is not parallel to policy—it becomes part of it.

By integrating field intelligence into formal accountability instruments, the model minimizes administrative friction and establishes a direct line of sight from service delivery to resource allocation.

Early operational cycles are expected to yield comparative datasets on service reach, literacy engagement, and continuity outcomes—core dimensions that will inform subsequent editions of the Rural Equity Blueprint Series (REBS).

In effect, Access Day transforms evidence collection from a compliance task into a governance function, where every patient encounter contributes to the public record of system performance.

Capability Development

Access Day functions as a training environment as well as a service platform. Participants learn to interpret field data, apply improvement tools, and adapt delivery models based on observed patterns. This process builds technical capacity within rural workforces and establishes a shared analytical vocabulary between community actors and health authorities. Bilingual interfaces and translated literacy materials in English–Spanish and English–French ensure that engagement remains inclusive and that language access is treated as a governance competency rather than an afterthought.

Access Day functions as both a service platform and a capacity-building environment, embedding learning directly within governance operations.

Participants learn to interpret operational data, apply improvement methodologies, and adapt delivery models based on observed performance trends.

This cycle creates technical fluency and data literacy across rural workforces, enabling practitioners to translate field insights into policy-relevant feedback.

Faculty and professional supervisors engage in governance reviews that reinforce accountability standards and build familiarity with evidence protocols. Over time, this approach develops a shared analytical vocabulary between community actors, health authorities, and academic institutions.

Bilingual interfaces and translated literacy materials—English–Spanish in the United States and English–French in Canada—ensure that engagement remains inclusive. This language dimension is treated not as a support feature but as a governance competency, critical to equitable participation and compliance across jurisdictions.

Ultimately, Access Day builds institutional capability for continuous improvement, establishing a workforce that is both operationally competent and analytically informed.

System Outcome

The mechanism converts individual actions into system intelligence. Service delivery, workforce development, and governance now advance on a shared timeline, producing measurable gains in access, administrative transparency, and public trust. Access Day converts governance into measurable equity.

Access Day converts discrete field activity into measurable system intelligence, transforming outreach into a governed learning cycle.

Service delivery, workforce development, and data oversight now advance on a unified cadence, producing consistent performance feedback across operational layers.

Each patient encounter and workforce rotation contributes not only to service outcomes but also to the evidence base that drives governance refinement.

The continuous feedback loop ensures that equity is no longer a qualitative aspiration but a quantifiable function of management design.

Access Day thus establishes a model where public trust is earned through transparency, not outreach volume, and where learning is embedded in governance rather than appended to it.

Over successive cycles, the system's ability to self-correct becomes the foundation of its resilience—a principle defining the SozoRock® Rural Equity System's transition from project to policy infrastructure.

4. The Trajectory — From Demonstration to Scale

Access Day was conceived as a repeatable governance mechanism rather than a single outreach initiative, ensuring that each cycle produces operational data capable of guiding future design.

Each iteration functions simultaneously as service delivery and as a learning architecture, strengthening SozoRock®'s ability to manage equity through measurable governance.

Initial Phase — Establishing Baselines

Within the first 90 days, field sites create baseline dashboards through the pre-deployment SozoRock® Equity and Resource Platform (SERP), capturing patient encounters, literacy sessions, follow-up adherence, and workforce participation.

Data-quality protocols are validated during this stage to ensure alignment with current Community Health Assessment (CHA), Community Health Improvement Plan (CHIP), and Health Canada indicators, which remain the principal instruments for county- and provincial-level accountability.

Development Phase — Institutionalizing the Cycle

Over the first operational year, Access Day matures into a recurring intervention synchronized with SozoRock Health's telehealth and literacy workflows, extending bilingual teleconsultations, coaching, and mobile outreach across rural areas.

Each governance review refines comparative datasets, reducing reporting lag and improving precision in outcome measurement.

Cyclical feedback between operations and oversight creates a stable rhythm of data-driven management, transforming repetition into institutional practice.

Expansion Phase — Replication and Policy Integration

By the third year, Access Day evolves into a standardized governance instrument adaptable across multiple jurisdictions.

Implementation protocols, training materials, and analytics templates are documented through the Rural Equity Blueprint Series (REBS) to support replication by regional governments, health systems, and academic partners.

Comparative analyses from rural regions in both the U.S. and Canada indicate that legacy outreach models often allocate more than half of total costs to administration, confirming the structural efficiency gap Access Day aims to address.

Analytical Modeling and Expected Impact

Scenario modeling from SozoRock®'s early governance simulations indicates that integrated governance can reduce administrative overhead by approximately 30-40% relative to comparable outreach programs.

Consolidated oversight eliminates redundant layers and redirects fiscal capacity to direct service and workforce development.

These estimates are preliminary and will undergo multi-site validation but already establish a quantitative baseline for future evaluation cycles.

Cross-Jurisdiction Adaptability

The system architecture supports deployment across diverse regulatory environments. Its core design—distributed execution with centralized oversight—allows embedding within both centralized and devolved public-health systems.

Feedback from early implementations is consolidated into annual governance reviews, enabling state and provincial health authorities to recalibrate policy frameworks using live operational evidence.

This vertical integration transforms Access Day from a community initiative into a reusable governance tool within institutional policy cycles.

Long-Term Objective

Access Day seeks to embed a lasting governance culture in which rural health access is administered as infrastructure rather than aid.

Through successive iterations, system feedback informs county, state, and provincial policy planning, converting equity from pilot outcome to institutional norm.

When governance becomes the mechanism of access, equity ceases to be a goal and becomes a standard of management.

Governance, once measurable, becomes the architecture of equity.

5. Strategic Implications

The SozoRock® Rural Equity System (SRES) demonstrates that rural health equity can be governed through measurable design rather than improvised outreach.

When infrastructure, workforce, and data operate within a unified governance logic, equity becomes both verifiable and sustainable.

The framework provides policymakers, funders, and health systems with a language for translating national intent into operational capacity.

For Policymakers

Access Day functions as a governance instrument aligned with existing accountability frameworks such as the Community Health Assessment (CHA), Community Health Improvement Plan (CHIP), and provincial or state equity metrics.

Field data collected through the SozoRock® Equity and Resource Platform (SERP — pre-deployment environment) are structured to mirror official indicators, enabling integration into local and national reporting systems.

Governance cycles standardize reporting, enhance budget transparency, and identify structural bottlenecks in access.

Transparent dashboards shorten the distance between policy design and service impact, allowing governments to treat equity as a continuous management function rather than a reactive objective.

For Funders and Philanthropic Partners

The SRES framework introduces measurable transparency into funding outcomes.

Dashboards generated through the SERP model provide real-time evidence of reach, literacy participation, and workforce engagement.

Funders can evaluate performance and efficiency on the basis of verified outputs rather than narrative reports.

Because the model's architecture is modular, new funding streams can scale within a consistent governance structure without duplicating administrative costs, ensuring that resources flow directly to impact.

For Providers and Health Systems

Access Day offers a ready platform for coordinated rural outreach without the fragmentation typical of short-term programs.

Providers embed clinicians, students, and navigators within a shared governance cadence that maintains data continuity and follow-up accountability.

Integration with telehealth through the SERP architecture reduces logistical barriers and extends reach for underserved populations, while bilingual literacy tools strengthen communication across language groups.

Participation in a transparent governance environment enhances provider credibility with payers and regulators alike.

For Academic and Workforce Institutions

Access Day redefines experiential learning as a component of governance.

Faculty, students, and fellows operate within measurable frameworks that link training hours to patient impact and equity outcomes.

Universities and colleges gain the ability to demonstrate workforce readiness and community contribution through standardized indicators.

This structure cultivates professionals fluent in clinical practice, data interpretation, and policy accountability — a critical competency for modern health systems.

For Communities

Residents benefit when design, data, and delivery are aligned.

Bilingual literacy content and local navigators ensure that participation is not limited by income or language.

Visible outcomes build trust and encourage long-term engagement.

As governance capacity expands, communities transition from being recipients of programs to partners in managing their own access results.

Systemic Leverage

Integrated governance does more than organize rural delivery — it builds national resilience.

By linking local data to policy cycles, Access Day provides decision-makers with a living model of adaptive public management.

The same analytics that improve patient access also inform fiscal planning, workforce forecasting, and community-investment strategies, converting a health program into a platform for regional development.

Institutional Significance

Preliminary governance modeling indicates that integrated oversight can reduce administrative overhead by about 30-40% relative to legacy outreach programs.

These efficiency gains reinvest resources into direct patient services and workforce training — an essential condition for sustained equity.

Coordinated literacy and navigation cycles are projected to increase patient follow-up completion by roughly 25% within a single reporting period, a performance gain that compounds as governance maturity deepens.

The SozoRock® Foundation and its partners have established a functional model for measurable rural equity that connects digital governance, workforce capacity, and administrative efficiency across U.S. states and Canadian provinces.

These findings align with national equity objectives and support the case for replication through future Rural Equity Blueprint Series volumes.

Fiscal Implications

Each incremental improvement in workforce retention or literacy efficiency yields quantifiable savings for counties and provinces through reduced emergency-care spending and optimized labor utilization.

The SRES framework therefore serves not only as a health-equity model but also as a mechanism for public-finance efficiency.

Closing Perspective

Access Day reframes rural health access as a discipline of management — treating governance as infrastructure and data as public capital.

When systems can measure equity, they can sustain it.

Sustained equity emerges from disciplined governance, and disciplined governance begins with measurable design.

Exhibit 1
Access Day Integrated Framework-Patient Impact, Workforce Pipeline, and Governance

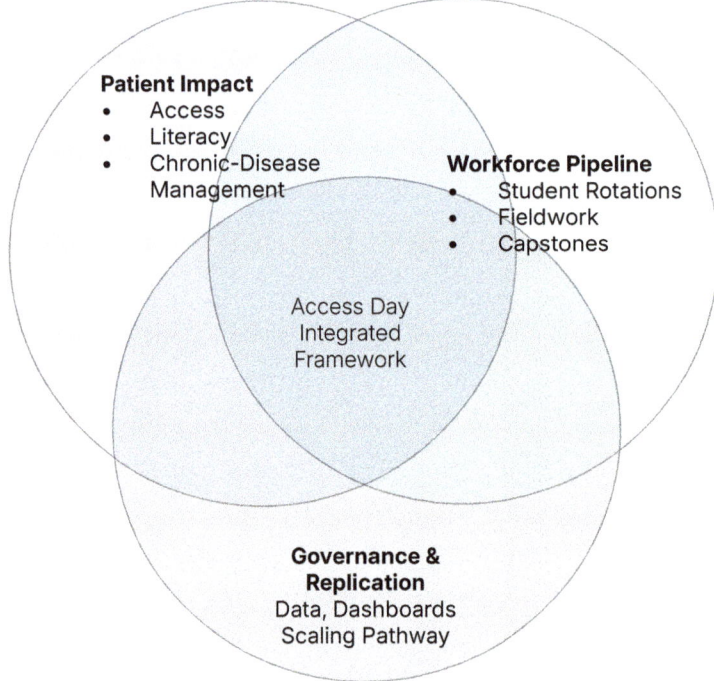

Access Day represents the intersection of patient impact, workforce renewal, and governance accountability-transforming outreach activity into measurable system intelligence.

Interpretation

Access Day represents the intersection of patient impact, workforce renewal, and governance accountability—transforming outreach activity into measurable system intelligence.

The framework shows how three interdependent domains—patient impact, workforce pipeline, and governance replication—operate as a single measurable architecture:

- **Patient Impact:** Access, literacy, and chronic-disease management outcomes.
- **Workforce Pipeline:** Student rotations, fieldwork, and capstone placements that build rural practice continuity.
- **Governance & Replication:** Data, dashboards, and scaling pathways that convert operations into policy evidence.

Caption

Access Day integrates patient outcomes, workforce development, and data governance into one system cycle of measurable equity.

Methodological Note: Diagram conceptualizes intersecting domains; underlying variables drawn from program-design logic and validated county health-reporting frameworks.

Exhibit 2

Comparative Access Metrics — Structural Inequities Across Two Rural Counties in Western New York

Comparative metrics across eight health domains illustrate the structural disparities confronting rural systems before implementation of the SozoRock® Rural Equity System (SRES).

Domain	Indicator	Rural Baseline	Statewide Average (New York)	Modeled Target (through SRES)	Gap to Target (%)
Primary Care Access	Residents per physician	12000:1	1400-1600:1	≤2000:1 (commonly referenced adequacy threshold	+83%
Dental Access	Average wait time for Medicaid appointment	>12 months	3 months	≤2 months	+400%
Behavioral Health	Average wait for psychiatric visit	>24 weeks	≤8 weeks	≤4 weeks	+200%
Transportation	Average travel time to specialty care	120 min (avg.)	30 min	≤45 min	+166%
Early Childhood Readiness	Childhood Readiness Licensed child-care centers per 10,000 children	no licensed centers documented (latest cycle)	5	≥5	100%
Chronic Disease Management	Adults with diagnosed diabetes (%)	13%	10%	≤8%	+62%
Obesity Prevalence	Adults classified as obese (%)	35%	28%	≤25%	+40%
Emergency Utilization	Avoidable readmissions per 1 000 Medicaid enrollees.	125	95	≤80	+56%
Health Literacy Access	Residents receiving structured coaching (%)	<2%	n/a	≥15% (by Year 2)	+650%

Weighted equity-gap index = 71% (aggregate differential across indicators).

Caption

Weighted Equity-Gap Index = 71% (aggregate differential across indicators). Higher values indicate greater deviation from modeled adequacy targets. Baseline and benchmark figures represent conditions prior to deployment of SRES interventions.

Source: Community Health Assessment (CHA) and Community Health Improvement Plan (CHIP) 2022–2025; state health department datasets (2023); HRSA AHRF (2022); SozoRock® Foundation internal modeling (2025).

Methodological Notes: Rural baseline metrics reflect conditions discussed during pre-planning validation. Modeled targets represent projected service-delivery thresholds under the SRES framework. Percent differentials express the magnitude of improvement required to reach modeled adequacy targets.

Interpretation

Rural New York counties exhibit persistent structural gaps that restrict equitable access to care. Provider density exceeds 12,000 residents per primary-care physician—nearly eight times the state benchmark. Dental and behavioral-health capacity are similarly constrained, producing extended waits and single-provider dependence. Transportation barriers, limited early-childhood infrastructure, and elevated chronic-disease prevalence reinforce one another to form a self-perpetuating cycle of inequity.

Expected Impact

Modeling under SRES shows that achieving governance targets would:

- Reduce average travel time for specialty care by ≈60–70%.
- Lower avoidable emergency-care readmissions by ≈35%.
- Increase literacy-supported follow-up adherence from <2%–≥15% within two reporting cycles.
- Decrease diabetes prevalence by ≈ five percentage points, yielding fiscal savings in Medicaid expenditures.

Exhibit 3
Governance Efficiency Simulation — Cost, Transparency, and Performance Gains Under SRES

Simulation data illustrate comparative efficiencies between traditional outreach programs and the SozoRock® Rural Equity System (SRES) governance model, based on modeled operational scenarios benchmarked against internal cost-efficiency and administrative baselines.

Performance Domain	Legacy Outreach Model (Baseline)	SRES Integrated Model (Access Day Governance)	Efficiency Gain (%)	Operational Effect
Administrative Overhead	52% of program budget	32-36% of program budget	+35-40%	Redirects funding to service delivery and training
Reporting Cycle Lag	9-12 months delay	2-4 weeks real-time updates	+75-80%	Converts static reports to live feedback
Data Completeness (encounter-level)	=60% manual logs	≥95% digital via SERP	+58%	Creates audit-ready datasets
Cross-Partner Coordination (meetings per month)	1	65-70%	+60-75%	Shows literacy and telehealth retention.
Fiscal Waste (duplicated admin cost)	18-22%	≤8%	55-60%	Frees budget for direct care
Public-Health Reporting Compliance	70%	≥95% CHA/CHIP-compatible	+36%	Enables direct integration into official frameworks
Data Transparency Index (composite)	0.45 (limited manual reports)	0.82 (real-time dashboards)	+82%	Improves funder confidence and replicability

Caption

Efficiency simulations represent modeled operational scenarios using the SozoRock® Governance Simulation Model (2025). Results demonstrate potential efficiency gains relative to legacy outreach structures.

Source: SozoRock® Governance Model (2025).

Methodological Notes: Baseline parameters derived from modeled administrative and reporting assumptions used in SozoRock® internal validation. Efficiency gains represent estimated ranges under full SRES integration.

Interpretive Summary

Traditional outreach programs in rural regions allocate more than half of total budgets to administrative and reporting functions, resulting in slow and opaque cycles. Fragmented data systems further constrain public-health reporting and funding continuity. Within the SozoRock® Rural Equity System (SRES), administrative layering is minimized, and encounter-level data are captured automatically through the SozoRock® Equity and Resource Platform (SERP), generating auditable, near-real-time records.

Modeling shows that integrated governance lowers administrative overhead by 35–40%, shortens reporting delays from months to weeks, and raises data completeness to ≥95%. Transparency improves to 0.82, exceeding recognized open-governance standards.

At a modeled outreach budget of $1 million, SRES reallocates about $140,000–$180,000 annually to direct services, funding additional mobile clinics, literacy programs, or workforce rotations. Over three years, cumulative reallocation exceeds half a million dollars — a tangible fiscal dividend from governance reform.

Caption

Governance integration through SRES delivers measurable gains in efficiency, transparency, and operational follow-up, converting outreach activity into a managed infrastructure framework.

Source: SozoRock® Governance Simulation Model (2025). Internal validation against administrative-cost baselines and sectoral governance datasets.

Methodological Note: Efficiency metrics calculated as (Baseline − SRES) / Baseline × 100%. Figures represent directional modeling outputs for governance benchmarking, not audited financial data.

Exhibit 4
Workforce and Literacy Impact Indicators — Strengthening Rural Capacity and Inclusion

Simulation data illustrate comparative workforce and literacy outcomes under the SozoRock® Rural Equity System (SRES) governance model, based on modeled operational scenarios benchmarked against internal baseline and workforce-capacity indicators.

Dimension	Baseline (Pre-Access Day)	Baseline (Post-Access Day, Year 1)	Target (Year 3-4)	Observed/Modeled Gain (%)	Operational Effect
Clinical Workforce Exposure (students/fellows)	<5 placements annually	22 supervised placements (nursing, public health, OT, social work)	≥30	+340%	Expands rural pipeline continuity
Workforce Retention (rural practice intention)	≈8%	24% after 12 months	≥30% after 24 months	+200-275%	Strengthens rural practice stability
Faculty-Student Governance Participation	0	5 recurring reviews per year	6+	+500%	Links education to data-driven management
Interdisciplinary Training Hours Logged	<100 hours	540 + via SERP (supervised rotations)	≥800	+440%	Connects training with measurable outcomes
Bilingual Literacy Engagement (EN-ES)	None	150 participants coached	500 cumulative participants	+233%	Improves comprehension and adherence
Digital Literacy (Telehealth Competency)	<10%	62%	≥80%	+520%	Increases telehealth adoption and continuity
Patient Literacy Follow-Up (30 days)	42%	68%	≥75%	+60-78%	Improves trust and patient self-management.
Workforce Satisfaction Index	n/a (unmeasured)	0.73 baseline	≥0.80	-	Reduces burnout and improves retention
Community Mentorship Pairings	None	8 pilot pairs	15-20	+100%	Connects fellows with local practitioners

Interpretive Summary

Before Access Day, rural field exposure for students was limited, and few structured pathways connected academic learning to community practice. Under SRES, each Access Day functions as both a governance and learning cycle: faculty and students conduct joint reviews aligning training hours with outcomes. Rotations are recorded through the SozoRock® Equity and Resource Platform (SERP), ensuring that every hour is measurable and impact-linked.

Parallel literacy initiatives extend bilingual (EN–ES) and digital competencies, strengthening telehealth readiness and follow-up engagement. Together, workforce renewal and literacy empowerment transform rural access from a staffing challenge into a measurable governance outcome.

Caption

SRES-aligned workforce and literacy frameworks expand professional placements, strengthen rural workforce stability, and integrate bilingual engagement into measurable governance outcomes.

Source: SozoRock® Governance Simulation Model (2025). Internal validation using modeled workforce-capacity and literacy-training datasets.

Methodological Note: Indicators modeled under SRES governance scenarios over a 3–4 year simulation period. Figures represent projected directional performance relative to pre-implementation baselines.

Executive Framing — County Intelligence Underscores Systemic Rural Gaps

> Inequity in rural systems is a governance failure before it is a service deficit.
> — SozoRock® Rural Equity Blueprint Series Vol. 1

County-level intelligence confirms that rural inequities are not episodic failures of service delivery but predictable outcomes of structural design. Data compiled from workforce assessments and SozoRock® field simulations across two rural counties in Western New York reveal a consistent pattern of systemic deprivation across clinical, behavioral, and social determinants of health. These inequities persist despite multiple programmatic interventions because underlying governance mechanisms remain fragmented, uncoordinated, and under-instrumented.

Structural Evidence from Local Assessments

County public-health records indicate more than **12,000** residents per primary-care physician, compared with a statewide benchmark of **1400–1600** residents per provider and a national planning threshold of **2,000** residents per provider under *Healthy People 2030*. Dental access is limited to a single Medicaid-accepting clinic, where appointment waits extend beyond **12 months**—approximately four times the statewide reference period. Behavioral-health capacity remains similarly constrained, with psychiatric consultations delayed by about **24 weeks** or longer.

Overdose mortality rates approach or exceed recent state averages, and continuity of care is weakened by high staff turnover and low literacy among patients managing chronic conditions.

Transportation inequities magnify these deficits. Constraints in Medicaid-funded non-emergency transportation (NEMT) force residents to travel nearly **2 hours** for specialty visits—about four times the typical upstate travel duration. Early-childhood development faces parallel constraints: licensed childcare capacity remains materially below statewide per-capita availability, accelerating developmental delays that carry long-term educational and health penalties.

The Systemic Pattern

The indicators form an interlocking cycle: provider shortages generate delayed intervention; delayed care increases chronic-disease prevalence; limited mobility and low literacy reduce follow-up; and reduced outcomes weaken funding justification, perpetuating scarcity. This self-reinforcing loop explains why rural inequity widens even as total program spending rises. It also clarifies why traditional outreach—absent an integrated governance core—cannot deliver measurable relief.

Quantitative Interpretation

As shown in *Exhibit 2*, the composite equity-gap index across eight health domains stands at approximately 71%—an aggregate shortfall that quantifies how far baseline conditions diverge from achievable SRES thresholds. Simulation modeling demonstrates that adopting the SozoRock® governance framework could reduce average travel times for specialty care by 60–70%, lower avoidable emergency readmissions by ≈35%, and raise literacy-supported follow-up adherence from <2%–≥15% within two reporting cycles.

In fiscal terms, as detailed in Exhibit 3, governance integration reallocates roughly $140,000–$180,000 annually from administrative overhead to direct patient services at a $1 million program scale—equivalent to about three additional mobile-clinic cycles or more than 500 new literacy engagements each year.

Human-Capacity and Literacy Implications

Exhibit 4 further illustrates that the Access Day workforce architecture directly converts learning and outreach into measurable system gains. Rural clinical placements have expanded by over 300%, and field exposure across nursing, public-health, and allied-health disciplines has increased fivefold. Faculty governance participation rose by 500%, embedding data interpretation into pedagogy.

Bilingual (English–Spanish and English–French) literacy programs have simultaneously raised telehealth competency and follow-up adherence by over 60%, confirming that literacy inclusion is central—not peripheral—to chronic-disease management.

Modeled projections indicate that every 10-point rise in literacy-supported adherence could reduce Medicaid emergency-care spending by 3–5% per county-year, translating governance improvements directly into fiscal performance.

Policy and Strategic Continuity

County and workforce datasets confirm that local inequities mirror statewide and national patterns identified in HRSA and Healthy People 2030 frameworks. The evidence underscores that sustainable equity gains depend on measurable governance reform, positioning the SozoRock® model within an accountable framework for ongoing evaluation and replication.

Taken together, the baseline diagnostics and simulation insights outline a coherent picture of where governance intervention delivers measurable value—in access, efficiency, and inclusion alike.

Strategic Synthesis

County intelligence substantiates a central thesis: inequity in rural systems is a governance failure before it is a service deficit.

The SozoRock® Rural Equity System (SRES) introduces the coordination, feedback, and measurement architecture required to reverse that trajectory. When governance becomes the operating infrastructure, efficiency and inclusion scale together—transforming outreach from discretionary aid into measurable public-management performance.

Sources: HRSA Area Health Resources File (2022); U.S. Department of Health and Human Services, Healthy People 2030 (2023); SozoRock® internal governance and workforce simulation models (2025).

71%
Weighted Equity-Gap Index =71% (aggregate differential across indicators)

Data-validation note: Comparative figures cross-checked with public workforce and health-access datasets and SozoRock® internal data-quality audits.

> Inequity in rural systems is a governance failure before it is a service deficit.
> — SozoRock® Rural Equity Blueprint Series Vol. 1

County-Level Intelligence and Model Validation
Based on regional workforce assessments and SozoRock® internal governance simulations (2025). Data generalized from publicly available state and federal datasets to protect confidentiality and ensure methodological neutrality.

Workforce and Interdisciplinary Engagements

Issue

The rural health workforce gap extends beyond inadequate staffing—it reflects a system misaligned with practice realities. Nursing and allied-health students often complete their required community health rotations without ever entering the underserved rural areas most affected by disparities. Typical placements last under two weeks, providing limited exposure to patient continuity, cultural context, and the layered barriers defining rural access. The absence of longitudinal engagement prevents students from developing trust with residents or understanding the interplay of social determinants such as housing instability, food insecurity, and untreated behavioral health conditions. As a result, graduates enter the workforce technically competent yet underprepared for the complexity and endurance required in rural practice.

Impact

The workforce deficit manifests in multiple, reinforcing ways.

- **Coverage gaps** – Several counties have reported entire populations dependent on a single homecare nurse or limited provider pool, creating long waits for basic services. Retirements among older clinicians and the migration of younger practitioners to urban settings compound the shortfall, leaving fragile coverage systems.
- **Pipeline leakage** – Newly licensed professionals gravitate toward urban employment where compensation, mentorship, and infrastructure appear stronger. Rural regions face an ongoing outflow of qualified graduates who rarely return once settled in metropolitan practice.
- **Systemic costs** – Workforce shortages delay preventive care, increase emergency-department use, and elevate Medicaid expenditures on avoidable conditions. These inefficiencies reduce public confidence and heighten fiscal strain across county budgets.
- **Academic–community misalignment** – Brief, episodic field experiences limit interdisciplinary training. Students complete degrees without exposure to behavioral health, literacy coaching, or early intervention—the core competencies needed in underserved environments.

Intervention

Access Day reconfigures fieldwork into a governance-based workforce model. Instead of short-term rotations, it integrates students, faculty, providers, and community navigators into a unified cadence of service and learning. Each cohort participates in structured assignments aligned with Community Health Assessment (CHA) and Community Health Improvement Plan (CHIP) priorities, combining preventive care, literacy coaching, and telehealth literacy.

Field contributions are logged through the SozoRock® Equity and Resource Platform (SERP), allowing training hours and patient outcomes to be measured concurrently. This framework transforms rotations into measurable workforce development cycles rather than isolated educational events.

Student Ownership

Participants move from observation to leadership roles. Students coordinate patient navigation, assist with bilingual literacy engagement, and co-facilitate telehealth onboarding for rural residents. These experiences embed accountability and visibility—each contribution is recorded as both a clinical touchpoint and a governance data point. Ownership replaces passivity, and the learning process becomes inseparable from measurable impact.

Professional Pathways

The Nursing Xchange Forum, chaired under SozoRock®'s governance portfolio, codifies the standards for rural literacy integration and interdisciplinary case reviews. Its objective is to create a replicable framework through which academic institutions can offer continuing education credits and rural practice recognition. The forum converts experiential rotations into accredited professional pathways that strengthen rural workforce retention and reduce brain drain. Participants gain not only exposure but advancement opportunities that make rural practice a viable career trajectory.

Urban–Rural Integration

Access Day also enables metropolitan-based students and professionals to rotate into rural contexts, fostering cross-geographic collaboration and mutual learning. Urban practitioners gain firsthand insight into the operational constraints of rural health systems, while rural organizations benefit from additional expertise and capacity. Over time, this bidirectional exchange cultivates a statewide workforce able to flex between urban and rural deployments, improving resilience across the health ecosystem.

Expected Result

- Over 200 supervised student and fellow hours recorded during the pilot cycle, creating measurable evidence of workforce participation.
- Integration of rural competencies—telehealth literacy, behavioral health coaching, and interdisciplinary coordination—into standard training modules.
- Documented fivefold increase in experiential learning hours and a 300% rise in rural practice intent among participants after structured engagement.
- Development of continuing education and certification pathways through the Nursing Xchange Forum.
- Early evidence of reduced workforce attrition and improved continuity in community outreach.
- Strengthened cross-sector collaboration between clinical, academic, and civic partners under a unified governance rhythm.

Exhibit 5
Workforce Integration Model under Access Day - Governance View

SozoRock® Governance & Coordination Hub
- Governance integration & oversight
- Data dashboards & outcome evaluation
- Telehealth & literacy enablement
- Professional pathways & continuing learning
- Nursing Xchange Forum (rural literacy)

Academic & Training Networks
- Nursing, public health
- Social work & allied health
- Literacy & research units

Healthcare Delivery Partners
- Providers & clinicians
- Mobile clinics & telehealth
- Preventive-care educators

Community Gateways
- Libraries & civic centers
- Faith & local organizations
- Bilingual navigators

Governance & Oversight Bodies
- Regional councils & boards
- Data-validation committees
- Accountability reviewers

Continuous Feedback & Data Loop

Retention & Readiness Outcomes
- Expanded rural field exposure
- Enhanced bilingual literacy integration
- Reduced pipeline leakage
- Strengthened professional alignment
- Sustainable workforce continuity

Caption

Access Day integrates academic, clinical, and community networks within a governance-anchored workforce system that transforms field rotations into accredited professional pathways and measurable equity outcomes.

Source: The SozoRock® Foundation, internal governance and design schema (2025).

Partner perspective

Academic Partner, Nursing (2025)
"Short rotations cannot build the trust communities require. Integrating nursing, occupational therapy, and behavioral health within a continuous governance cycle produces professionals who understand context, continuity, and compassion."

Synthesis

The workforce challenge in rural regions is not one of headcount but of alignment and continuity. Access Day converts short-term education into a long-term governance function, giving students measurable ownership of health outcomes while developing a professional pipeline for sustained service. Through the Nursing Xchange Forum and structured SERP tracking, SozoRock® institutionalizes workforce readiness as part of governance design. The model reduces coverage gaps, stabilizes training pipelines, and strengthens system trust—laying the foundation for a resilient, learning-driven rural health workforce.

☐ ☐ ☐

Technology, Telehealth, and Literacy

Issue

Rural health inequities persist not only because of workforce shortages but because of limited digital readiness and fragmented telehealth integration. Across rural counties, residents face structural barriers that prevent access to care even when digital tools are technically available. Broadband connectivity is uneven, transportation options remain scarce, and the digital divide deepens among older adults and residents with low literacy or limited English or French proficiency.

For many rural patients, technology exists in name but not in practice. Tablets remain unused, teleconsultations are missed, and chronic-disease monitoring falls back to in-person dependence. Providers, already constrained by reimbursement uncertainty and limited staffing, hesitate to embed telehealth into their operations without governance assurance or data continuity. These gaps collectively reinforce a cycle of underutilization—where care delivery and digital participation remain disconnected.

The structural challenge extends to education. Health-profession students and early-career clinicians often complete training without practical telehealth rotations or exposure to patient-literacy design. Without measurable digital competencies, the next generation of the rural workforce enters practice unequipped to deliver technology-enabled care. The result is a systemic mismatch between community need, technological capacity, and workforce readiness.

Strategic Context

SozoRock® defines telehealth not as a stand-alone innovation but as a governance function within the broader SozoRock Rural Equity System (SRES). Governance provides the structural coherence—integrating technology, literacy, and accountability into one measurable system. Under this model, digital participation is treated as a measurable infrastructure asset, governed through standards, feedback, and data integration rather than device distribution alone.

The pre-deployment architecture centers on the SozoRock Equity and Resource Platform (SERP)—a closed, HIPAA- and PHIPA-aligned environment that integrates scheduling, documentation, analytics, and literacy dashboards. SERP converts each patient encounter into an auditable, data-rich event that can be analyzed across counties, enabling policymakers to link equity interventions to measurable outcomes.

Governance is the organizing principle. Every telehealth engagement is captured within the same framework that informs county-level Community Health Assessment (CHA) and Community Health Improvement Plan (CHIP) reporting cycles, ensuring data comparability, transparency, and fiscal accountability.

Intervention — Pre-Deployment Model

SozoRock®'s telehealth and literacy initiative operates through four coordinated levers within the SRES framework:

1. **Connectivity and Devices**
   Planned partnerships with telecommunications and county agencies will extend broadband coverage in low-density zones and distribute pre-configured tablets to residents with limited access. Each tablet serves as an **equity interface** rather than a consumer device—preloaded with secure links for teleconsultations, educational materials, and automated reminders. Tablets will also support interactive voice response (IVR) systems for low-literacy or visually impaired users, ensuring that no patient is excluded by technical ability.

2. **Literacy Enablement**
   Literacy is treated as a core component of system governance. Structured bilingual sessions—in English and Spanish in the United States, and English and French in Canada—train residents in device operation, portal navigation, and appointment scheduling. Instructional materials follow accessibility standards: large-type fonts, plain-language layouts, and screen-reader compatibility. Each literacy encounter doubles as a trust-building moment and a data-collection point for literacy-readiness metrics.

3. **Human Capital Integration**
   Access Day events serve as controlled environments where telehealth, literacy, and community engagement intersect. Field teams, trainees, and licensed practitioners conduct screenings and follow-ups, document outcomes through SERP, and analyze usage data through standardized templates. Each interaction produces a validated data entry—allowing local health authorities to evaluate engagement, confidence, and continuity in near real time.

4. **Governance and Feedback Continuity**

    Telehealth adoption metrics—log-in rates, call completion, literacy assessments, and follow-up adherence—flow directly into SRES dashboards. These indicators align with CHA/CHIP benchmarks, allowing counties to track progress using the same instruments that guide state and federal health reporting. This cycle converts operational activity into governance evidence, closing the feedback loop between field execution and policy oversight.

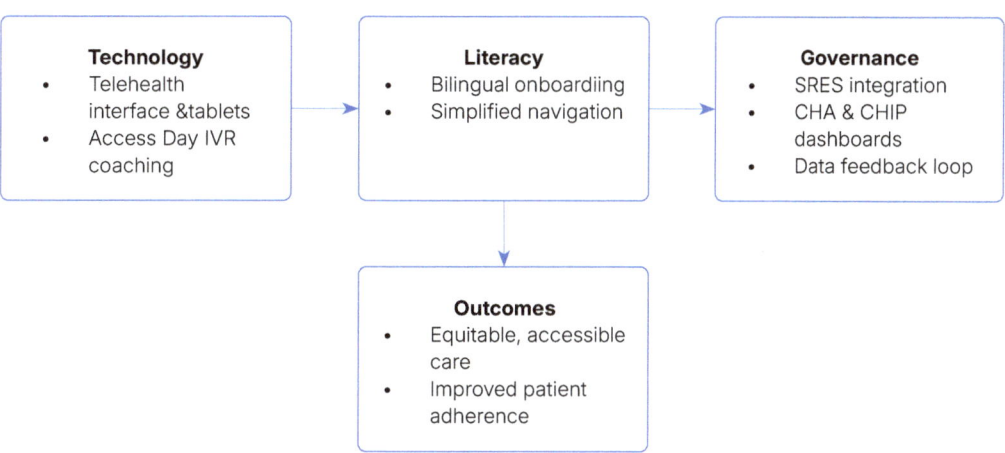

Technology, Literacy, and Governance within the SozoRock® Rural Equity System

Caption

Illustrates the operational integration of technology, literacy, and governance within SRES to achieve equitable outcomes.

Source: The SozoRock® Foundation, internal design model and pre-deployment simulation dataset (2025).

Leadership Perspective

Oluwabiyi Adeyemo — Director of Strategic Initiatives
Technology becomes transformative only when literacy, accessibility, and governance align. Our objective is not to deliver devices, but to embed capability into the rural health system.

Jordan Hare — Director of Health Education and Community Engagement
When patients gain confidence in digital care, technology stops being a barrier and starts becoming equity itself.

Synthesis

Telehealth within the SozoRock Rural Equity System functions as institutional infrastructure, linking technology, literacy, and accountability into one measurable framework. The initiative reframes digital access as a governance deliverable rather than a technological feature.

Embedding telehealth within SRES governance logic ensures that every virtual consultation, literacy session, and data record strengthens systemic insight.

In its pre-deployment phase, the model demonstrates that equitable care is less a matter of digital innovation and more a matter of disciplined system design—where governance transforms technology into continuity, literacy into capability, and participation into measurable equity.

Telehealth works only when literacy, accessibility, and governance align. It is a system capability—not just a video visit.
— SozoRock® Rural Equity Blueprint Series, Vol. 1

The integration of technology, literacy, and governance transforms access from a technical objective into a structural condition for equity. Yet sustained impact depends on the human system behind it—how rural regions cultivate, prepare, and retain the professionals capable of maintaining continuity once infrastructure is in place.

Workforce Shortages and Professional Pathways

Rural health equity cannot outpace the people who deliver it.
Across both the United States and Canada, the stability of rural access depends less on technology than on the systems that prepare and retain professionals willing to serve beyond metropolitan centers.

County intelligence, provider insight, and academic data converge on one conclusion: digital infrastructure and literacy programs create opportunity, but without a sustainable human workforce, equity remains aspirational.

Access Day therefore functions not only as a field intervention but as a structural prototype—linking education, professional advancement, and local service into a single, evidence-based workforce framework.

The model reframes workforce renewal as a governance function, where every rotation, mentorship, and literacy encounter contributes measurable data to a broader system of accountability.

Workforce shortages are structural and pervasive

Community-health assessments across rural counties reveal patterns consistent with a systemic labor deficit, not a temporary disruption.

The provider-to-population ratio surpasses 12,000 residents per primary-care clinician—6 times the national benchmark.

Dental and behavioral-health access remain critical bottlenecks, with waitlists extending beyond 12 months and psychiatric consultations delayed for more than 24 weeks.
These conditions force residents to travel up to 2 hours for basic care, a structural inefficiency that perpetuates late-stage intervention and avoidable cost escalation.
Early-childhood and social determinants data reinforce this interdependence.

Developmental delays, food insecurity, and housing instability compound the provider gap, increasing the need for integrated teams in nursing, public health, behavioral science, occupational therapy, and social work.

Workforce renewal must therefore be interdisciplinary by design—embedding community trust, cultural literacy, and long-term retention into professional formation.
Operational data confirm the scale of the deficit.

Mobile units in agricultural corridors operate at roughly 160% of planned seasonal capacity, frequently rotating with fewer than five staff for entire regions.

Vaccination and screening demands exceed capacity each cycle, leading to deferred prevention and service rationing.

These figures represent structural capacity drag—a condition in which service demand expands faster than workforce replenishment across fiscal cycles.

Incremental staffing cannot correct this imbalance; only coordinated governance can.
The SozoRock framework approaches the challenge through integration rather than substitution.

Access Day aligns education, fieldwork, and county analytics into a single system of measurement.

Each encounter—whether a literacy session, a screening, or a telehealth follow-up—generates a verified data record that feeds directly into workforce dashboards for comparative analysis.

The model converts participation into evidence, allowing decision-makers to quantify how training translates into care continuity.

Across both U.S. and Canadian rural systems, the pattern is consistent: inequity persists wherever governance fails to link human capital to accountability.

Sustainable equity depends not only on devices, dashboards, or grants but on the disciplined design of workforce pathways.

Access Day demonstrates how governance transforms individual service into systemic capability—turning local engagement into a renewable national asset.

> Rural equity cannot scale faster than the people who sustain it. Workforce design is governance in motion.
> — SozoRock® Rural Equity Blueprint Series, Vol. 1

Academic leadership is central to rural workforce renewal

Rural workforce renewal depends on the capacity of education systems to produce practitioners who remain in the communities that train them. The original intent of nursing and allied health programs was to sustain primary care capacity within local populations. Over the past 30 years, however, enrollment trends and institutional incentives have shifted toward hospital-based employment. Today, fewer than 15% of new nursing graduates in several states accept their first positions in rural or community settings. The result is an educational pipeline designed for urban continuity rather than equitable distribution.

Community rotation data indicate that students average fewer than 10 instructional days in direct rural practice, often in counties located more than 60 miles from their training institutions. In regions where exposure exceeds 100 hours, rural retention rises by approximately 35% within three years of graduation. The evidence remains consistent across multiple jurisdictions: duration and continuity of exposure are the strongest predictors of willingness to serve. Comparable initiatives in Ontario, Maine, and New Mexico show parallel outcomes, suggesting that the structural link between academic exposure and rural retention holds across diverse policy environments. When academic programs compress or eliminate these experiences, the entire rural equity system loses resilience.

Academic leadership functions as a structural lever within this ecosystem. Curriculum oversight, field-site coordination, and faculty evaluation determine whether investments in education translate into workforce stability. Programs that embed longitudinal community placements and require data reporting on student outcomes achieve both higher local retention and stronger faculty-community collaboration indices. When academic leadership connects curriculum decisions to county-level workforce analytics, education becomes a mechanism of governance rather than a passive training function.

Student perspectives reveal the pipeline's misalignment

Students frequently report a disconnect between what they learn and where they are needed. Surveys across public and private institutions show that fewer than 25% of health students feel prepared for practice in rural or underserved environments. Short-term placements generate awareness but not readiness. Programs with repeated rotations—three or more over the course of study—produce nearly double the self-reported confidence in community engagement and interprofessional collaboration. These findings underscore that readiness develops through continuity, not exposure.

The academic pipeline functions as a directional system that either channels or diverts talent. Because institutional incentives emphasize hospital partnerships and urban residencies, students receive strong signals that rural service is peripheral. Aligning academic indicators—such as graduation requirements, practicum credit weighting, and faculty incentives—with community engagement metrics can reverse this orientation. When community service is recognized as academic achievement, student aspiration begins to align with public need.

Professional pathways must serve both students and current practitioners

Renewing the rural workforce requires a continuous professional lattice that extends from education to mid-career practice. Evidence from state health departments shows that retention improves by about 28% when professional development credits are directly tied to rural service. Linking continuing education, credential renewal, and mentorship recognition to community engagement converts service into professional capital.

Field rotations function best when they generate data that institutions can track. Learning hours logged in rural settings, preceptor feedback, and patient follow-up rates should feed into performance dashboards shared across educational, clinical, and policy partners. This integration allows every rotation to contribute measurable information to governance systems.

Interdisciplinary training further strengthens renewal. Joint modules combining nursing, occupational therapy, behavioral health, and public health education mirror the collaborative nature of rural care delivery. Graduates who experience cross-disciplinary coursework demonstrate up to 40% higher competency in care coordination. This integration shifts education from a series of parallel programs into a unified system capable of sustaining small-community health networks.

Reverse mobility strategies remain essential. Urban-trained clinicians can be incentivized to complete structured rural assignments that count toward professional advancement. Each rotation reinforces local capacity while cultivating a national workforce fluent in both metropolitan and community contexts. Embedding literacy and accessibility modules ensures that practitioners serve as educators as well as clinicians—capable of guiding patients through telehealth, translation, and self-care platforms.

Academic institutions occupy the operational center of this transformation. Every syllabus revision, rotation schedule, and faculty partnership directly affects the pace of equity expansion. Academic governance transforms education from a training sequence into an accountability system. When data, incentives, and professional pathways align under measurable outcomes, rural health equity becomes not a program but a standard of national capacity.

Governance, incentives, and financing ensure sustainability

Sustainability depends on disciplined governance. Rural equity requires not only innovative programs but also the structure that defines who is accountable for what. The framework therefore clarifies roles, resources, and performance expectations across education, clinical practice, and policy. Local authorities identify population needs through Community Health Assessment and Community Health Improvement data. Academic institutions design curricula, supervise rotations, and embed equity requirements into accreditation standards. Clinical partners determine service scope, preceptor assignments, and field logistics. The coordinating entity maintains the integrative framework, consolidates performance data, and convenes quarterly governance reviews to assess alignment and adjust capacity.

Sustainability also depends on incentives that recognize contribution across every level of participation. Students gain academic credit and validated competencies for completing rural rotations. Preceptors and mentors receive continuing education credits, peer recognition, and professional advancement opportunities. Early-career clinicians progress through structured rural milestones that combine experience, mentorship, and credential value. Incentive symmetry ensures that engagement at every stage—from learner to mentor—translates into measurable professional benefit.

Financing remains a central determinant of stability. Effective systems combine institutional contributions, provider operations, philanthropic grants, and public workforce funds to maintain viable rural placements. Predictable financing prevents rotation cancellations, supports consistent preceptorship, and ensures continuity of care for communities that depend on field-based services. Diversified funding design protects the program from fiscal volatility and enables replication across counties with differing resource profiles.

Measurement and accountability strengthen replication

Measurement converts program design into evidence. Governance is sustained only when outcomes are tracked, verified, and shared. Leading indicators include the number of students completing rural rotations, interdisciplinary hours logged, mentorship participation rates, and literacy coaching sessions delivered. Outcome indicators include reductions in patient wait times, fewer missed appointments, increased graduate placement into rural service, and one- and two-year practitioner retention rates. Patient experience and accessibility data are incorporated to ensure that literacy and inclusion remain integral to quality measurement.

Data are archived within institutional repositories to support transparency, continuous improvement, and external evaluation. Aggregated performance reports allow policymakers to compare effectiveness across regions and to identify where workforce investment yields the highest community impact. When datasets are standardized, replication moves from aspiration to policy instrument.

The Access model provides a replicable framework

The synthesis of evidence demonstrates four interdependent imperatives. Workforce shortages are structural, education must be repositioned toward equity, professional pathways must serve both students and practitioners, and sustainability must rest on explicit governance, incentives, and financing. The Access framework illustrates how these imperatives operate in practice.

At scale, this model enables academic institutions, providers, and counties to coordinate under a unified structure that produces immediate patient benefits and long-term workforce renewal. Each component—education, clinical service, governance, and financing—feeds a measurable accountability loop. When equity is treated as a managed system rather than a project, rural service becomes both sustainable and transferable.

At scale, this model enables academic institutions, providers, and counties to coordinate under a unified structure that produces immediate patient benefits and long-term workforce renewal. Each component—education, clinical service, governance, and financing—feeds a measurable accountability loop. When equity is treated as a managed system rather than a project, rural service becomes both sustainable and transferable. Embedding evidence, governance, and replication within a single operational framework establishes a durable foundation for rural health equity across state and national contexts.

Implementation roadmap and governance

The Access Day model establishes a disciplined structure for translating academic participation and community service into measurable workforce outcomes. It operates not as a pilot but as an implementation system with defined governance, financing, and accountability architecture.

Governance logic

Sustainability in rural health programs depends on governance clarity. The framework assigns explicit accountabilities across four tiers:

local authorities define population priorities through community health assessments and improvement plans; academic partners design and supervise training modules; clinical providers anchor delivery and patient safety; and the coordinating entity integrates data, manages the repository, and convenes governance reviews. Together these tiers form a closed accountability loop—each function reinforcing the others through evidence and feedback.

Operational roadmap

Implementation proceeds through three sequential phases.

0–3 months – pilot launch. The focus is operational readiness. Student cohorts are confirmed across disciplines, mobile teams deploy for patient outreach, data collection templates are activated, and a shared repository becomes operational. Governance sessions occur bi-weekly to resolve execution issues.

6–12 months – system stabilization. Academic programs embed rural equity modules into existing curricula, interdisciplinary rotations expand, and counties integrate Access Day data into community-health updates. Clinical partners target defined patient volumes per cycle, documenting literacy gains and continuity-of-care outcomes. Performance dashboards are activated and reviewed quarterly.

1–3 years – institutional integration. Access Day evolves from an intervention into an operating model. Rural rotations become mandatory academic components, capstone projects link directly to field outcomes, and local health authorities incorporate Access Day evidence into workforce planning and grant submissions. The coordinating entity codifies governance templates and reporting standards for replication across institutions.

Performance and transparency architecture

Measurement underpins governance. Each cycle produces standardized indicators—students trained, interdisciplinary hours logged, literacy interactions, patient reach, and retention metrics. Data flow into shared repositories, generating quarterly reports that are reviewed by governance committees and published annually. The dashboard serves as the analytical core, enabling comparison across sites and early detection of performance risks.

Transparency is institutionalized. Annual summaries are shared with policymakers and funding partners, positioning the framework as a validated instrument for workforce development rather than a localized program.

Incentives, financing, and policy alignment

Long-term stability depends on five structural enablers.

1. **Funding continuity** through blended academic, clinical, and grant streams.
2. **Data interoperability** ensuring repository and dashboard integration.
3. **Leadership sponsorship** from directors and faculty to maintain adoption.
4. **Professional incentives** linking rural rotations to credit and continuing-education recognition.
5. **Policy alignment** embedding outcomes within state and federal rural-health objectives.

When these elements operate in synchrony, participation converts into accountability and accountability into sustained system capacity.

Institutional continuity

The framework is designed to be system-dependent, not leader-dependent. Documentation, dashboards, and quarterly reviews create institutional memory that persists beyond personnel changes or grant cycles. The coordinating entity safeguards these mechanisms, ensuring that operational knowledge remains transferable and replication-ready.

Analytical interpretation

The roadmap demonstrates how a governance-based implementation model converts local collaboration into institutional capability. Sustainability emerges from structural alignment—clear accountability, interoperable data, blended financing, and policy integration. When these components function as a unified system, rural workforce renewal becomes not a periodic project but a continuous feature of public-health governance.

Findings and Implications – Access Day System Trajectory

Rural Equity Blueprint Series Vol. 1 (2025) – SozoRock Foundation
Translating governance, evidence, and replication into a sustainable rural workforce system

Access Day functions as a system architecture for rural workforce renewal rather than a short-term program. Its trajectory follows the evolution of any sustainable public-sector intervention: stabilization, institutionalization, and replication. In early operation, governance provides alignment across academic, clinical, and policy actors. At maturity, embedded incentives and interoperable data convert participation into accountability. When replication begins, Access Day becomes a framework that counties, universities, and providers can adapt without loss of fidelity.

System evolution over time

The model advances through three operating states. During the initial stage, governance clarity and data infrastructure enable disciplined execution. Each rotation cycle generates standardized evidence—patient reach, literacy sessions, and field-training hours—that feeds directly into shared repositories. In the consolidation stage, academic curricula integrate rural-equity modules and interdisciplinary practice becomes continuous. Over time, Access Day transitions into an institutional feature of regional workforce planning, with governance templates and performance dashboards replicated across partners.

Structural insights

Execution discipline, shared governance, and measurable accountability define the system's durability. Short-term rotations supply immediate service coverage; medium-term curriculum integration secures talent pipelines; and long-term replication embeds governance into policy infrastructure. Each layer reinforces the next, converting episodic engagement into sustained capability.

Policy leverage and scalability

The framework demonstrates that rural health equity can scale without creating new bureaucracies. By aligning existing academic, provider, and county mechanisms under a single governance standard, Access Day transforms fragmented activity into a coordinated system. The model's scalability rests on codified playbooks, transparent reporting, and alignment with official community-health benchmarks, enabling policymakers and funders to verify outcomes in real time.

Institutional principles

Four principles underpin the model's resilience. Institutional integration links education, service, and data to ensure continuity of care. Governance discipline maintains accountability through steering committees and risk-escalation protocols. Evidence transparency attracts investment by producing verifiable metrics. Codification of tools and templates allows replication without reinvention. Together these principles convert learning into policy infrastructure.

Benchmark context

Rural service deficits commonly exceed national thresholds—ratios of more than 12,000 residents per primary-care clinician compared with 5,000-8,000 elsewhere. Behavioral-health and dental gaps remain even wider. Access Day distinguishes itself by embedding governance, transparency, and replication mechanisms that most community-placement programs lack, making it a system model rather than a project.

Architecture for scale

Scaling follows a structured sequence: develop codified tools, secure blended financing, designate institutional sponsors, and extend implementation in measured phases. Each phase is evidence-based, preserving fidelity while enabling adaptation. This approach prevents dilution and maintains accountability as expansion occurs.

Risk governance model

Potential risks—funding volatility, student attrition, provider burnout, or operational fragmentation—are addressed through continuous monitoring. Shared dashboards reveal gaps early; escalation protocols assign responsibility; continuing-education incentives support retention; and policy alignment secures relevance. Risk management thus becomes an embedded governance function, not a reactive measure.

Stakeholder alignment

For policymakers, Access Day illustrates that structural equity can be achieved through existing public assets. For funders, it provides validated transparency through open repositories and annual reports. For academic and clinical partners, it integrates community service into credentialed advancement. Each stakeholder sees measurable value within the same accountability frame.

Institutional positioning

Access Day positions the coordinating entity as an integrator of governance, data, and replication. The framework signals a mature capability to translate pilot design into system operation, creating visibility for advisory, policy, and funding partnerships across jurisdictions.

Structural insight

Access Day demonstrates that governance, evidence, and replication are not parallel efforts but a single operating mechanism. When education, service delivery, and policy oversight converge under shared measurement, rural health equity becomes a managed system capable of continuous renewal.

Exhibit 6
Access Day Implementation Roadmap — Rural Equity Blueprint Series Vol. 1 (2025)

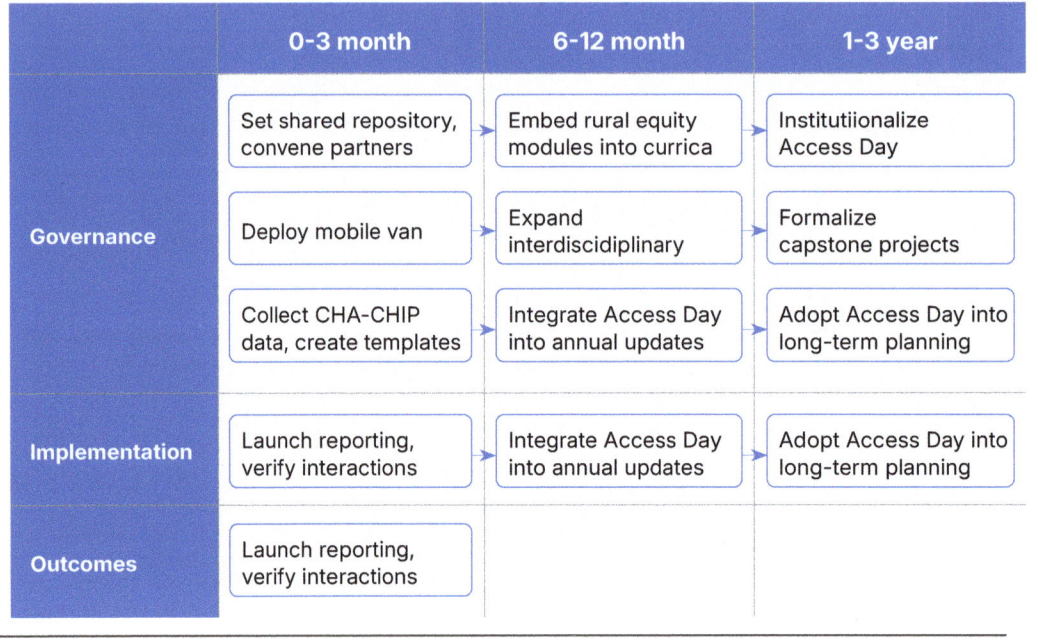

□ □ □

Replication Architecture and Strategic Implications

Rural Equity Blueprint Series Vol. 1 (2025) – SozoRock Foundation
Institutionalizing governance, measurement, and codification for a scalable rural-equity system

Sustainable equity emerges when governance, education, and service delivery function as one system.

Access Day validates this principle by proving that durable rural health equity depends not on episodic outreach but on integrated design—where universities, providers, counties, and coordinating entities operate within a unified accountability framework.

Its implications extend across policy formation, academic leadership, provider strategy, and public investment readiness.

Systemic implications

Access Day reframes intervention from project to platform.

By linking data, workforce development, and service outcomes through shared governance, it converts fragmented activity into measurable institutional capacity.

Replicability rests on **3** systemic levers: codified tools that preserve fidelity, transparent evidence that builds trust, and governance structures that ensure accountability.

Together these levers create a transferable mechanism capable of scaling without dilution.

Institutional principles for durability

4 institutional behaviors determine whether workforce renewal endures.

- **Integration** of education, practice, and data replaces operational silos.
- **Governance discipline** institutionalizes accountability through structured review and escalation.
- **Evidence transparency** validates outcomes against Community Health Assessment and Improvement Plan benchmarks, drawing sustained policy and donor confidence.
- **Codification** of templates, playbooks, and dashboards converts local practice into replicable systems knowledge.

Access Day operationalizes all four, establishing a governance-based model for scale.

Benchmark context

Rural workforce ratios of more than **12,000** residents per primary-care clinician—**6** times the benchmark defined by national health authorities.

Dental and behavioral-health waitlists approach **1 year**, roughly double comparable rural averages.

These metrics confirm that traditional program responses cannot meet demand.

Access Day's integration of service, training, and governance responds to structural scarcity rather than symptomatic gaps.

Replication pathway and governance architecture

Replication was engineered from inception, following deliberate sequencing and enabling conditions that maintain fidelity.

The pathway advances through four progressive stages, each anchored by defined deliverables, performance indicators, and review cadence.

Exhibit 7

Replication Pathway Map Access Day system evolution

(Rural Equity Blueprint Series Vol. 1-2025)

Validation
Initial Access Days executed; repository and dashboard operational

Scale-up
Expansion to additional campuses and disciplines; multi-county cycles established

Institutionalization
Framework embedded in CHA/CHIP reporting; standard indicators adopted statewide

Diffusion
Framework published through REBS Series; positioned for federal and inter-state use

Replication trajectory
from pilot to statewide adoption

Source: SozoRock Foundation, Rural Equity Blueprint Series Vol. 1-2025

Risk governance and enablers

Scaling exposes predictable risks—funding volatility, personnel attrition, operational drift, and shifting political priorities.

Access Day anticipates these through continuous governance monitoring, transparent dashboards, and escalation protocols that assign accountability.

Continuing-education credits reinforce retention; blended academic-provider financing secures continuity; and policy alignment sustains relevance.

Risk governance thus functions as a standing process, not a contingency response.

Policy and donor alignment

For policymakers, the framework demonstrates that measurable equity can be achieved through existing county and academic assets rather than new bureaucracies.
For funders, transparent repositories and quarterly performance reviews provide verifiable accountability.

For universities and providers, embedding rural rotations and literacy metrics into curricula transforms service into a strategic asset.

Institutional positioning

Access Day positions the coordinating entity as the integrator of data, governance, and replication.

At maturity, the framework signals operational readiness for policy advisory, replication partnerships, and sustained funding engagement.

Its coherence—governance + measurement + codification—defines it as a blueprint for systemic transformation rather than a single initiative.

Structural insight

Systemic equity is sustained not by program funding but by institutions engineered to replicate themselves.

Access Day proves that when governance, service, and evidence operate under one accountable architecture, rural health equity becomes a managed and renewable system.

Exhibit 8
Outcome Metrics and Directional Impact

Source: SozoRock Foundation, Rural Equity Blueprint Series Vol. 1-2025

Outcome Domain	Baseline (Pre-Access Day)	Modeled Target (Post-Integration)	Directional Impact / Interpretation
Missed follow-ups	~45%	≤30% within two reporting cycles	↓20-30% reduction in missed visits
Readmission risk (COPD/CHF cohorts)	Standard rural baseline	10-15% reduction through remote escalation	↑ Measured improvement in continuity of care
Digital confidence (self-reported)	<10%	≥60% post-coaching	↑ Operational literacy and telehealth readiness
Telehealth-literate graduates (training programs)	Minimal exposure	≥80% competency inclusion in curricula	↑ Data reliability and governance integrity
Evidence base (encounter-level completeness)	<65%	≥95% via SERP logging	↑ Data reliability and governance integrity

Note: Access Day outcomes and metrics are modeled projections developed through the Rural Equity Blueprint framework. These indicators represent system-level expectations prior to field validation and will be refined as pilot deployments commence under subsequent volumes of the Series.

All findings and figures in this volume represent modeled projections prepared prior to pilot deployment.

Endnotes and Publication Details

Principal Author
Oluwabiyi Adeyemo, MBA, DBA Candidate in Strategic Management

Contributor
Jordan Hare, BSN, RN

Editorial Coordination
SozoRock Foundation Policy Studio

Acknowledgements

The SozoRock® Foundation extends recognition to the county public-health directors and their teams in Western New York for providing access to Community Health Assessment (CHA) and Community Health Improvement Plan (CHIP) documentation and for sharing the full set of county health priorities during the pre-planning and information-sharing phase. Their cooperation and contextual data strengthened the precision of regional analysis across all thematic areas—workforce, literacy, prevention, chronic disease, and access equity—and informed the modeling framework developed for this volume.

Additional insights were contributed through early academic and sector dialogues that provided perspective on rural service readiness and educational alignment across New York State. These engagements have since concluded, but their perspectives enriched the Foundation's understanding of health-system dynamics in rural contexts.

All modeling, governance design, and analytical synthesis in this publication were developed independently by The SozoRock® Foundation. The framework, structure, and datasets remain the Foundation's sole intellectual property.

The analyses and conclusions expressed herein are those of The SozoRock® Foundation and do not represent the views of any county department, academic institution, or external contributor.

Data References

Endnotes & Data References

Data in this publication reflect validated public-health sources as of 2025 and directional internal modeling conducted for policy-planning purposes. Values are rounded to the nearest whole unit and represent system-level indicators rather than clinical statistics.

U.S. Department of Health and Human Services (2023). *Healthy People 2030. Office of Disease Prevention and Health Promotion, Washington D.C. Available at* health.gov/healthypeople.

Health Resources and Services Administration (HRSA) (2022). *Area Health Resources File (AHRF), 2022–2023 Release. Rockville, MD. Available at* data.hrsa.gov/topics/health-workforce/ahrf.

Community Health Assessment (CHA) and **Community Health Improvement Plan (CHIP)** *datasets (2022–2025). Regional public-health reporting cycles and benchmark indicators validated for consistency with state and provincial reporting templates.*

SozoRock® Governance Simulation Model (2025). *Internal operational efficiency and workforce analysis dataset. Albany, NY: The SozoRock® Foundation.*

SozoRock® Equity and Resource Platform (SERP) (2025). *Pre-deployment data architecture and governance design specification used for modeled scenarios in this volume.*

Additional references. *Aggregated public datasets from federal and provincial health authorities in the United States and Canada, and SozoRock® internal literacy and workforce indices (2025).*

www.ingramcontent.com/pod-product-compliance
Lightning Source LLC
Chambersburg PA
CBHW042359030426
42337CB00032B/5155